How to Become a Former Asthmatic

How to Become a Former Asthmatic

PAUL SORVINO

William Morrow and Company, Inc.
New York

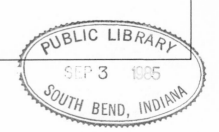

Library of Congress Cataloging in Publication Data

Sorvino, Paul.
How to become a former asthmatic.

Includes index.
1. Asthma—Treatment.   2. Breathing exercises.
I. Title.
RC591.S66   1985   616.2′38062   84-16528
ISBN 0-688-01220-5

Printed in the United States of America

4 5 6 7 8 9 10

BOOK DESIGN BY SUSAN HOOD

For Michael

Foreword

In his book *How to Become a Former Asthmatic,* Paul Sorvino, actor, operatic tenor, and Renaissance man, outlines breathing exercises that have helped him and many others overcome asthma. Asthma itself is difficult to define even for the physician. It is much easier to describe its manifestations: wheezing, a feeling of being out of breath, and coughing. These symptoms are worsened by exertion and anxiety. Although sometimes there is an identifiable allergic cause, frequently there is none. Many drugs have been employed in the treatment of asthma. Most commonly, these are medicines that open the breathing tubes or those which fight inflammation or allergy, such as cortisone. There is presently no *cure* for this disease, if, as Mr. Sorvino wonders, it even is a disease.

Using layman's terms, Mr. Sorvino describes a series of breathing exercises that are easy to follow. I can attest to this because I watched him take my then-fifteen-year-old son through them in fifteen minutes. I can also vouch for their efficacy. They work. But like any exercise or training program, discipline and repetition are required. Slow and steady wins the race.

Paul Sorvino is not naïve enough to believe his regimen is infallible. Nor is he out to suggest it replace the pediatrician, allergist, or chest specialist. I suggest you try Mr. Sorvino's exercises. You have nothing to lose but your asthma.

—CHARLES G. GARBACCIO, M.D.

Acknowledgments

With love to Harriet Strachstein

I wish to thank Adrienne Claiborne who first exposed me to the nuts and bolts of the writer's trade, Eric Weber for suggesting this book, and Bill Adler for helping me plan it.

My deepest gratitude goes to my extraordinary family, Mira, Amanda, Michael, and Lorraine. It is of course Lorraine's support, faith, and love that have made everything possible.

Contents

Foreword   7
Acknowledgments   9

PART I: Asthma   13
1. What Is Asthma?   15
2. What Can Be Done About Asthma?   22
3. Other Things to Do   42

PART II: My Story   45
4. How I Overcame Asthma   47
5. Michael's Asthma   58
6. More Games   66

PART III: Sharing the Exercises   71
7. Case Histories   73
8. You and Your Doctor   86

Index   93

PART I

Asthma

CHAPTER I

What Is Asthma?

If you were to go to a mirror now and watch yourself take the biggest breath you possibly could, you would notice a distinct raising of your chest and shoulders plus a stiffening of your entire upper body. You would also notice that you're not getting much air for your effort. I'm sure of this because in twenty years of watching, I've never seen an asthmatic breathe any other way.

Combine this inefficient breathing technique with the genetic predisposition (asthma runs in families) or a strong sensitivity to dust, pollen, animal dander, mold, or allergic reaction to certain foods—and you get the quick, shallow breathing pattern known as asthma.

What's happening is your body is reacting in an exaggerated way. Congestion (mucus) occurs in your bronchi, your sinus cavities, your overall breathing mechanism. The body panics from lack of oxygen and sends out a desperate message to breathe faster. Hence, the spasm.

This overreaction occurs in nine million people in America alone. It attacks young and old, rich and poor, weak and strong. It causes serious handicaps for its sufferers by aggravating other illnesses such as coronary disease (a number of people die every year from heart attacks brought on by the desperate force engendered by spasmodic, shallow breathing). It has plagued the human race for millennia and, as yet, medical science can offer no cure.

And I believe the reason it has found no cure is that asthma is not really a disease.

I know this is a radical statement. Doctors have always treated asthma as a serious disease and have traditionally prescribed strong medications to fight it. They deserve no blame for this. They have had no choice.

But in these pages I will support the belief that the spasm we're talking about is removable by other than medical means. The asthma itself is simply a disorder of the respiratory process. Something out of whack in a normally natural and productive sequence of events.

I base this belief on twenty years of experience in helping remove the disorder from myself, my son, and scores of others.

For the moment let's accept the idea that asthma is a mistaken breathing pattern, so that we can begin to think of it in terms of correction. That is really what this book is about. If it is successful for you, it will teach you to breathe all over again. And the way you breathe has everything to do with getting rid of the spasm. In this attempt, let's use an analogy for purposes of clarification: THE ANALOGY OF THE BALLOON.

If you enclose the bottom part of an empty balloon in your fist and try to blow it up, all you'll be able to do is inflate the neck—the smallest, narrowest part. But if you open your hand, the entire balloon will inflate, assuming you supply continuing and sufficient air pressure.

Now think of your lungs in relation to the balloon. By breathing high up in the chest area, you are duplicating the same constricted air-intake process as when the bottom part of the balloon was enclosed in a fist. The only area you're giving yourself are the "necks" of the lungs, i.e., the trachea, bronchial tubes, and bronchial spaces.

The large, capacious bottom sections of your lungs remain virtually unused. This doesn't become apparent unless you try to take a big breath, but it goes on all the time, whether you're aware of it or not.

What Is Experienced by an Asthmatic?

As you probably know too well, the spasm can begin with a cold, an allergy attack, or a stressful event of any kind. Stress in itself can cause powerful alterations in the most normal person's breathing function, and the attendant strong emotions, such as anger or fear, can create a greater need for oxygen in a hurry.

But however a spasm begins, it usually follows a predictable course. You become aware of a shortness of breath with growing congestion in your chest. You cough but produce nothing. As your breathing becomes more labored, your fear begins to mount. If the spasm is severe, you fear for your very existence. This nightmare scenario can last hours, days, months, years, or the rest of your life.

The doctor will usually give a shot of Adrenalin, perhaps followed by a series of medicines including antihistamines, antibiotics, bronchodilators such as Tedral, and in severe cases, a cortisone derivative such as Prednisone or Vanceril. Many asthmatics are forced to live permanently on these medicines. On cortisone-dependent children, the effect can be bizarre. They may not grow to normal height. Their bodies swell disfiguringly. Their emotions can be chaotic. I saw this in my son. Although he was only on cortisone for two weeks, he experienced such a hyperkinetic wildness that we began to fear he'd hurt himself by careening into the furniture.

I also saw these side effects at the children's asthmatic center in Ossining, New York. A number of the fifty or so children in residence there are cortisone dependent. Some have been brought to the center by ambulance. A few have brushed close to death.

I went there with my son, Michael, who was then four years old, to explain the exercise program that had cured us. Unfortunately, the time allotted was short, and the administrative atmosphere not really conducive to sharing this information, but at least we tried.

I remember working particularly hard with a ten-year-old girl who had almost died the week before. She was the height of a six-year-old and her face and body were markedly swollen. I was drawn to her because of the intelligence and yearning in her eyes. I gave her as much individual attention as I could, but with children her age, one session is not sufficient time in which to learn the exercise concepts. It remains a fond hope that somehow this marvelous child has found competent, loving attention and has regained her health.

Later in this book, I outline a system for teaching children effective breathing exercises that can eliminate the need for cortisone therapy. It was created by my son and me when he suffered his nearly lethal asthma attack three years ago. It has been elaborated on by my wife, Lorraine, whose contributions and dedication have been so helpful to Mike.

What Does It Do to You?

Asthma may not be a disease, but if you have it long enough, it will look and feel like one. Your chest can become distended from years of breathing too high. Cortisone may have caused your body to swell disfiguringly. Your constitution may be weakened—cortisone can play havoc with your system if taken for too long a time, or if you're taken off it too suddenly. Antibiotics over the long run can also kill the "good" germs in your body, setting you up for a massive infection. The bronchodilators may hurt the heart from years of pulse quickening. And, of course, cortisone can have a tragic effect on children by preventing them from reaching full height.

As a practical matter, asthma can be severe economically as well as physically. My life had been a history of frequent doctor bills, prescriptions, injections, and allergy testing, all costly and time consuming. Asthma also delayed the start of my opera career by at least twenty years—but more on that later.

There is the loss of work time from frequent bronchial infections and spasms. Some asthmatics move to other locales to escape indigenous allergens. But even if that works, it can be costly in terms of abandoned job opportunities; and the move can put undue stress on the rest of the family.

How Does It Feel?

Like you have just raced fifty yards at full speed, though all you've done is gotten up from your chair. You can't catch your breath, your chest is heaving, and you're coughing unproductively. Of course, people without asthma feel fine again within a few minutes. An asthmatic feels out of breath all the time.

It can make life lose its naturalness, for you and for those around you. Understandably, it's tough for them to pretend everything is fine while you stand there gasping for air. And reactions vary from individual to individual. One may take your dilemma as a burden and be angry about it, another may empathize and go through every difficult moment in your corner.

But since asthma isn't a heroic affliction like ulcers or heart trouble, i.e., caused by hard work or high-level decision making, it tends to make people contemptuous of you. They see it as "psychosomatic," and "all in your mind." What they are often thinking is, "You are causing everyone a great deal of aggravation, time, and trouble. Don't be an annoying weakling. You bring this on yourself."

The best thing you can do is reject this attitude right now and for the rest of your life.

I would like you to believe that there is no loss of dignity in having asthma. It doesn't matter one bit how you got it, or what psychological factors are helping maintain it. All that matters is how you are going to get rid of it. And get rid of it you can. Very soon. Perhaps before you finish reading this book.

CHAPTER II

What Can Be Done About Asthma?

The exercises you are going to learn in this chapter will be with you for the rest of your life. Take the time to learn them carefully without pressure of time or telephone. Allow at least an hour for the first session and try to make it as uninterrupted as possible. If you can't set aside this much time, start anyway. The sooner you start, the sooner you will be breathing freely. Also, it would be a good idea to reread this chapter through at least once before trying to execute the instructions. (Should you have any back, heart, or other problems, talk the exercises over with your doctor before trying them.) If at any time you are not sure of a particular technique, stop. Relax. Keep the book at your side and refer to it as often as necessary. Remember, this is neither a test nor a race. You have probably had asthma for a long time. It is a formidable opponent. Give yourself the chance to defeat it methodically and completely.

* * *

First, make sure you're not wearing any restrictive clothing. A good outfit for doing these exercises is a jogging suit or shorts and a T-shirt. The best outfit is nothing at all because you will need to see what your body is doing, especially above the waist.

Now take a chair (a regular kitchen chair will do) and position it in front of a mirror where you will be able to see your upper body while seated. You will also need a floor mat or carpet, and you will have all the necessary equipment.

The first part of the exercises is done lying comfortably on your back. Once in this position, place your hands at your sides at the bottom of your rib cage, thumbs pointed downward, fingers up.

Relax for a moment and prepare to enjoy what you are about to do.

- When you feel reasonably calm of body and spirit, start to take an easy breath with your mouth closed. Do this while mentally counting slowly to four. As you progress with the count you should begin to feel some pressure of the incoming air on your hands. If not, you are probably breathing too "high" in the chest area. Exhale. Relax.

    Think back to the analogy of the balloon. If you did not feel pressure on your hands, you were only using the "neck" of the balloon to inhale. This is simply a matter of habit, one you must break. You must retrain yourself to inhale deeply into the lungs without perceptibly raising your chest. (Raising your chest is all right if you do so before you take the breath; just be sure not to do so while you are inhaling.)

Try again. Inhale slowly through the nose with your mouth closed. This time try to mentally direct the flow of air to where your hands are placed. Take as much time as you need to learn this part of the exercise.

In fact, don't go on until you are sure that you understand it from a purely physical point of view. Remember, you must feel increasing pressure on your hands as you fill up the bottoms of both lungs. If you are doing this correctly you will also notice a slight expansion of the area just below the solar plexus. This is all to the good, for now you are employing the front part of the large muscle known as the diaphragm. It is worth pointing out that the so-called diaphragmatic breathing, as it is taught by most respiratory therapists, concentrates only on the expansion of this stomach area without recognizing the fundamental importance of the full side expansion of the upper body (below the rib cage) to ensure a total inflation of the lungs. When this partial technique is taught it produces only a slight improvement in inhalation capacity, but almost always causes tension in the body. This hampers the breathing of an asthmatic even further. But if you wish to try it, go right ahead. In my experience, when an asthmatic or anyone else does this, all that results is a strong, stiff abdomen within a few weeks. If you do the exercise correctly, however, the result will be a strong, flexible diaphragm with a much greater inhalation capacity.

To recap: hands at your sides . . . raise the sternum (chest) . . . inhale slowly through the nose while mentally counting to four . . . feel the pressure at your sides where your hands are placed . . . don't let the breastbone rise while you are breathing.

• When you have done this enough times to have mastered the sensation, you will have learned the inhalation portion of true diaphragmatic breathing. Now comes the second phase which is, appropriately enough, the exhalation. Here is where the diaphragm takes a very active role. The diaphragm is actually a muscle that extends from your stomach all the way around to your back. It controls the respiratory functions, but in an asthmatic, it is almost always weak from lack of use. Most people don't have to think about the function of the diaphragm, with the exception of singers and certain athletes. Our purpose as soon-to-be former asthmatics is to develop this muscle and bring it under conscious control. In doing this, however, we must take care not to confuse muscular effort with tension. Even at the greatest heights of muscular effort, such as in Olympic weightlifting, the accent in training is on relaxation. There is a body building phrase that cautions: "Train. Don't strain." Good motto for an asthmatic too.

On the other hand, relaxation does not mean flaccidity. Nothing will be accomplished if in the fear of becoming tense you do too little. With breathing exercises, as with any coordinated physical effort, the trick is always to find the productive middle ground. I would also add that when in doubt, do *something*.

With practice you will learn relaxation in breathing.

All right, now that you are reasonably sure you can take a large breath by expanding your lungs from their bottoms up, do just that, using the count of four. Now purse your lips firmly and exhale as if you were going to blow out a candle. The result should be a steady, controlled stream of air expelled to the count of four.* While exhaling, the front part of the diaphragm will naturally want to pull in somewhat. This is natural and necessary. Actually, it is the diaphragm that is giving you the force to produce the stream of air. It is the sensation of pulling up just under the breastbone, or sternum. The diaphragm here is performing a function that is exactly analogous to a bellows. If you compress the air chamber in a bellows, a controlled and powerful stream of air will result. The air is focused by a small opening at the mouth, and it is just this process that we want to copy.

If you are doing this comfortably, you have learned the basic exercise. Not as tough as you thought it would be, is it?

Let's practice it again. Chest up. Relax the stomach area (let it drop). Inhale, counting slowly to four until your hands are pressured outward and you feel your lungs reasonably full. Exhale, counting slowly to four with strongly pursed lips.

---

*It is important to purse the lips tightly. To test this, actually light a candle and blow out the flame at increasing distances. The tension produced in the lips by the attempt to blow out a flame two feet away is about right for the exercises.

• So far so good. Let's try a variation. Inhale on a count of four. Now exhale, but this time let the exhalation last as long as is comfortable for you. Continue to count until you exhaust the air in your lungs. In most cases, the exhalation will be longer than the inhalation. Either way, make note of it. I personally like to begin my exercises taking the same number of seconds in and out, sometimes building up to ten and ten, twelve and twelve, or whatever seems comfortable at the time. The important thing is to establish a rhythm for yourself that you can sustain for at least five minutes while you lie on the floor. You may wish to vary the seconds after the first minute or so. Feel free to do so. Try eight and eight. Six and six. Six and four. And so on. You're the boss.

Observe the fact that now you are beginning to deal with your affliction in an organized way.

So much for the floor portion of the exercise. No matter how long you have just spent learning it, from now on five minutes will be enough. After the first "training" session, your entire program will take less than fifteen minutes, once in the morning, once again at night.

By now you should be feeling a little better. If your breathing was labored when you began, you will probably feel a slight easing, almost the beginning of a sense of well-being. If not, don't worry, you will feel better soon enough. At this point you may want to cough. Don't be afraid; the coughing sensation is a direct result of the exercise and is extremely important. By now the mucus in your bronchial spaces is beginning to be acted upon by the force of air you have been creating. It is analogous to a mud-encrusted garden hose being cleared by a burst of strong water pressure. Chances are, if you do cough, it will be productive—a very different cough from the dry, frightened, and debilitating cough to which you are so accustomed.

At this point it would be wise to drink a big glass of water, since it is a very good expectorant. You should drink at least ten glasses a day. So drink up, cough up, and let's go on.

• Raise yourself from the floor and sit on the chair. By the way, this chair should be the right size for you. That is, it should allow your feet to reach the floor comfortably with your thighs and shins forming a right angle. Now place your hands, palms down, on your knees. Take another moment to relax. Begin the same exercises you just completed on the floor. Four and four, six and six, six and eight, etc. Chest up. Drop the abdominal muscles. Inhale through the nose, then exhale through the mouth against the pursed-lips pressure. If at any time you feel that you are not getting it right, stop. Try again. If you are not sure that you are filling your lungs from the bottoms up, put your hands on your sides as you did on the floor. You should again feel a graduating pressure as your lungs fill up. Do the exercises easily—without pushing—for at least ten minutes, or as long as it takes you to get a feel for them. They are as much art as science, and although they have a very specific effect as long as you do them reasonably well, their efficacy will improve as your coordination improves.

Now finish this portion of the exercise by reversing the count. If you have reached eight and eight, start switching back to, say, six and six, four and four, three and three, two and two, one and one. Now inhale and exhale through the mouth only. Accelerate forcefully until you sound like a speeding locomotive. Don't be embarrassed. This activity is seen and heard only by you and your asthma. If you get dizzy or feel lightheaded, don't be alarmed. It simply means that an excess of oxygen has reached your brain and you are hyperventilating. It is not dangerous. Just relax on the floor for a moment or two.

At this point, whether you know it or not, you are demonstrating to yourself that you can control your respiration. You are sending a message to your unconscious that you no longer wish your asthma to control you. Up to now, it has been a malevolent and mysterious adversary. No longer. You have penetrated the mystery and are methodically going about the business of removing the fear. When you were an infant you breathed in and out quite naturally. Between then and now something went haywire. You need not know the exact cause of this interruption of your natural breathing function in order to recapture it. It is enough to know that at one time you did it correctly and you are now, more or less, doing it correctly again.

To further concretize this process, take a good deep breath in the manner which you have just learned and say aloud, as you exhale, something like this: "I will no longer tolerate you, asthma. Go away! I have better things to do with my life than to carry you around with me." Say this several times a day. You will be surprised at the result. The great tenor Enrico Caruso could be heard through his dressing room door before every performance shouting repeatedly for someone to go away. When asked who had dared to trouble the eminent *divo,* Caruso replied, "No one. I holler at the little man in myself who says I cannot sing tonight." Caruso knew a great deal about the power of positive shouting.

• Now you are ready for the exercise with which you will end each session. It is called the Bellows. It is a powerful and condensed form of the exercise you have just learned but—and I stress this—it must be done *only* after the floor and chair portions are finished, due to the considerable amount of relaxation, coordination, and physical force it requires.

Sit erect on the chair with your hands placed comfortably on your knees. Take a deep breath (no counting needed) and begin your exhalation—but this time, start leaning forward from the waist very slowly. As you do this, consciously exert a steady pull on the front part of your diaphragm. This pulling in of the diaphragm should be in synchronization with the outward flow of air from your pursed lips. The movement should last about ten seconds, at the end of which your head should be close to your knees and you should have exhaled most of the air in your lungs. At this point you will attempt to push the remaining air out of your lungs by exerting even more inward force with the diaphragm and changing the position of your lips so that you can make a hissing sound through your teeth. Where before you have been trying to restrain the escaping air with pursed lips, you now will seek to express all remaining air by using this SSSSS sound, the noisier the better.

When you feel you have no more air to exhale, begin to rise from the waist. Inhale through the nose, slowly, mouth closed. It is a good idea to let the air resonate in the pharynx (that area just behind the uvula, the back of the throat) so that you can hear the intake of air. It will allow you to monitor the steadiness with which you are inhaling and will verify that you are actually taking the air into your lungs. This rising portion of the exercise should also be done very slowly. Remember of course to breathe from the bottom up, so to speak, allowing your sides below the rib cage to expand slowly and completely. As your upper body reaches the erect position you should be full of air. Be sure that during this movement you have not expanded the upper chest area or raised your shoulders.

When you arrive at the sensation that tells you no more air can be taken in, lean forward again from the waist—but this time, do it very quickly so that your head reaches between your knees in less than a second. As you push forward, exert a powerful inward force on your diaphragm area (just under the solar plexus) as if you were reacting to a sudden punch. If you are doing this correctly, the air will be rushing to escape—and it is at this time that the very strong pursed-lips position is extremely important. When your head is between your knees and you have exhaled most of the air, switch again to the hissing sound and force the last remaining bit of air from your lungs, even to the point of saliva escaping from your mouth. This usually happens at the end of the movement and helps to indicate that you are doing it correctly.

Now relax and sit up slowly. If you feel uncomfortable or lightheaded, just lie on the floor for a moment or two. You have now reached the end of your first workout. And I'd be willing to bet you are feeling much better. As you do these workouts, once in the morning, once at night, you will increase the number of Bellows you can do. Thus, at the end of each week, you can add one or two, depending on your age and general fitness. By the time you reach twelve Bellows, I can almost guarantee that you'll be free of the asthmatic spasm.

Here a caution is required. If you have heart disease, you must build up to the Bellows very slowly. If your condition is severe, I would advise you to skip it entirely. The floor and chair portions of the workout will give you enough benefit to improve your breathing permanently without the risk of straining yourself and causing more illness. If you are at an advanced age, I would make the same caution. If you have any doubt about the Bellows, show this book to your doctor and be guided by his advice.

Good health is a cumulative accomplishment. Even if you are in good health other than your asthma, you should not seek to accelerate the exercises before you are ready for them.

When to Do Your Exercises

It is my experience that the best time is in the morning and evening, preferably before or long after having eaten. It is difficult to move flexibly on a full stomach. But there are many opportunities during the day when you can do a mini form of the basic exercise. For a period of three or four months after my asthma was cured I would find myself walking the street breathing in through the nose and exhaling against slightly pursed lips to a varying count. It gets to be enjoyable after a time and the more oxygen your body can get in a day, the better you are going to feel.

If you have trouble learning the exercises correctly, don't despair. Keep at them. If you practice and refer to the instructions often enough, you will become proficient. I, personally, have never known anyone to be incapable of learning them. But, if in the learning process you become discouraged, break the exercises down into their parts, much as a pianist breaks down a piece of music—phrase by phrase and note by note. After countless repetitions familiarity is inevitable.

The fact is that vigorous, healthful breathing must become a way of life for you. You must enter it into your "muscle memory." Once you do, you will have at your disposal a weapon that can defeat your asthma permanently.

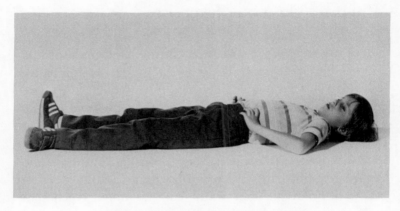

Mike is in proper floor position to begin.

Mike has already inhaled and is beginning forceful exhalation. Note that Mike uses the ''candle-blowing'' pursed-lips position.

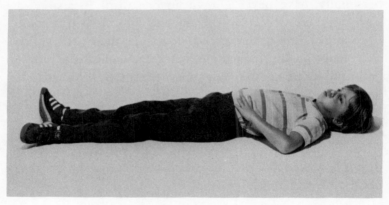

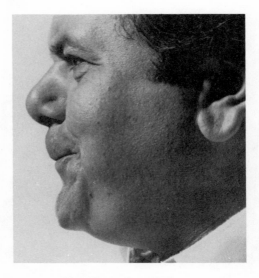

His old man's technique.

Notice that I use a position more
resembling that of a wind instrument player.

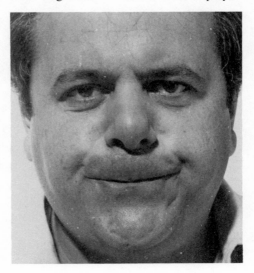

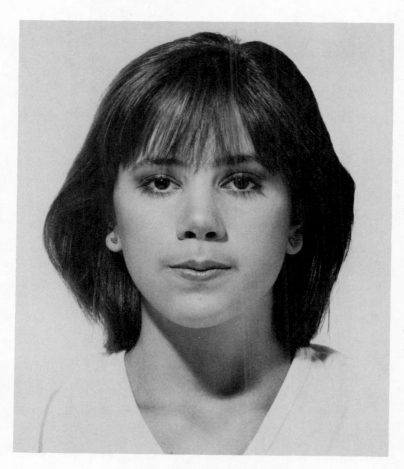

Mira's version.

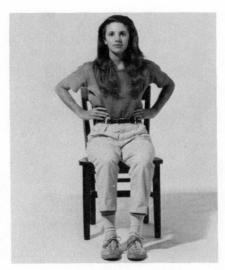

Amanda showing us proper hand
position to check inflow of air.

Amanda shows us the posture for
the chair portion.

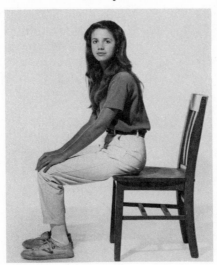

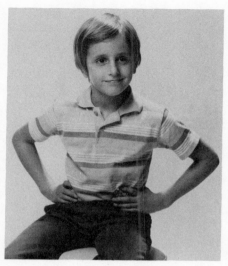

Mike begins his inhalation—
note position of hands and closed mouth.

Mike's lungs are filled. Note that his shoulders are not
raised but his middle is fully stretched.

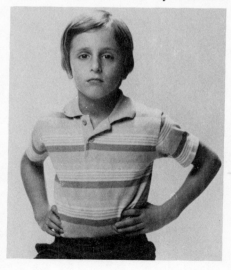

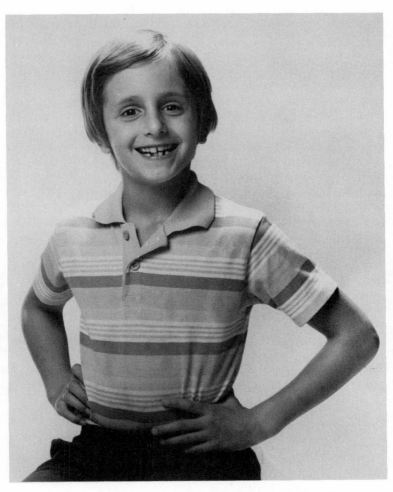

Mike had already exhaled before the camera could
catch it, but he wants to show us how good it felt.

Mira begins Bellow's forceful exhalation.

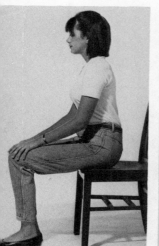 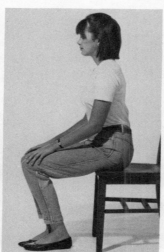 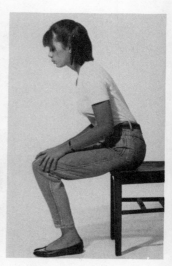

In the following series you will note that Mira's neck
does not bend as she leans forward.

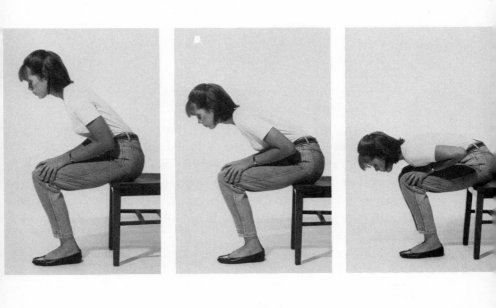

CHAPTER III

Other Things to Do

The information I am going to share with you now comes from the bits and pieces I have culled in the last twenty years that I have been free of asthma. Experiment with it as much as you can and, more importantly, develop and elaborate on the basic theme. Anything you discover to be effective might help others, so please write to me about it in care of the publishers.

The Punching Bag

This may seem extreme to you, or even silly. But there are a number of psychoanalysts who believe that patients who work out on a punching bag need fewer therapeutic sessions per week than those who don't. For myself, after hitting the light and heavy bags for even a few minutes, I feel better emotionally.

I suspect that it has to do with the basic hitting function, which is all but denied to modern man. In ancient times human beings were forced to use this technique just to get through the day. When attacked by enemies, human or otherwise, fists or clubs had to employed on a regular basis. Hunting entailed hitting or throwing. Even in more recent times, chopping firewood or rug beating demanded this function.

Thus, at the risk of oversimplifying, I would suggest that because we are denied the hitting function by modern society, we are also denied the "natural" method of releasing tension and potentially dangerous emotions. Although it has obvious value for society at large, the repression of anger and aggressive feelings in an individual can cause real emotional and physical illness. This bottling up of emotions is particularly harmful to an asthmatic. But using a punching bag is a sociologically acceptable form of hitting and a very good exercise in its own right.

I will never forget the answer an asthmatic boy gave me when I playfully asked him if he wanted to fight. He said, in a most knowing way, "If I wanted to fight, I wouldn't have asthma."

When you find yourself irritable and difficult to live with, go to the bag, picture your troubles, and punch away. You needn't tell anyone why—it's your business. A garage or basement is an adequate space and the expense is minimal. When I first tried the idea the whole family got into the act. One at a time we assaulted an old cushion with a long stick. After a few minutes there was a burst of laughter from all participants, including my seventy-two-year-old mother, who hit the thing harder than any of us.

Psychotherapy

The problem of repression leads to the question of whether psychotherapy is valuable in the treatment of asthma. While punching a bag tends to release bottled-up emotions, the deeper exploration of the effect of these emotions is best done with the help of an analyst.

If, given the genetic predisposition, asthma represents a chronic maladjustment to a once-threatening stimulus, it follows that we as adults can take the opportunity to correct that maladjustment. To find a better defense, or perhaps remove the defense entirely. Many of the problems we faced as children are no longer with us, but curiously, it is in the nature of human behavior to maintain and fortify a defensive structure once it is built.

For example, if you had a fault-finding parent, you will probably not take criticism easily in your adult life.

Psychotherapy can also help develop assertiveness, which is so important in the fight against asthma. This is particularly important because the condition of asthma itself encourages one to behave in passive, placating ways. When we have it, we tend to feel guilty and may end up habitually thanking those around us for putting up with us. It isn't a conscious response but one acquired out of a distinct need to lessen the emotional stress engendered by those whose patience we think we are straining.

PART II

My Story

CHAPTER IV

How I
Overcame Asthma

The first time I can remember having asthma was when I was ten years old. My mother and I had journeyed from our home in New York to California. She and my father were in the midst of marital difficulties that prompted her to leave. My brothers refused, but I, the youngest child, decided to go with her. I suppose, in a way, I was siding with her. It was a frightening and exhilarating experience all at the same time. We were "on the lam," and this appealed to my adventurous nature. We crossed the country in four days on a Greyhound bus and landed in Los Angeles with nothing but an old guitar and four dollars in Mama's purse.

A dear old lady by the name of Mrs. Gordon, who had been a friend of the family when we lived in Los Angeles the previous year, took us in as orphans of the storm.

As soon as we arrived I developed the spasm. I was put to bed for four days and doted on by my mother and Mrs. Gordon. My mother soon found a job as a practical nurse, and I was left in Mrs. Gordon's care during the day. It turned out to be a blessing. To entertain me, she began to tell the story of her journey to California many years before. She told me how in the 1870s, when she was a little girl, her family braved the cross-country trip in a Conestoga wagon all the way from "Ioway," as she called it. There was an old, rusted pistol up on a shelf that she used to let me play with while she fascinated me with tales of that wagon-train journey. The pistol was broken and of course unloaded, but I slipped it through my belt, put myself back on that wagon train with her, and imagined the most wonderful adventures.

The trip had been long and difficult and I loved every minute of it, begging her to not leave out the smallest detail. There were wild Indians and dangerous animals to contend with. There was bad weather and privations of every sort that "we" had to endure. When what she told me wasn't exciting enough, I would imagine myself doing all the things I knew that real cowboys did. Like ordering "sa'sparilla" in a tough saloon, as "Hoppy" would. Or singing my way into the sunset like The Lone Rider. What a marvelous way to get well. Ah reckon ah jes' rode outta mah asthma, Pardner.

The metaphoric conclusion is not merely in jest. Thirty-four years later I have come to understand that "Mother" Gordon, in her wise and loving way, was helping me romanticize what was surely a frightening experience for a ten-year-old boy—leaving my father and brothers three thousand miles behind.

With the innate skill of a practiced clinician she transferred my reality trip into a fantasy one, invoked my courage, and helped me do battle on my own terms with those fearsome immediate circumstances. That overwhelming experience, which could have been devastating, was transformed into a calming and strengthening adventure. She is surely long gone now, but over the years I have often thought of her with love and admiration for her generous wisdom and unique goodness.

But as the years went by, my asthma returned periodically. My family situation changed again when my father spirited me from California a year and a half after my mother and I had arrived at Mother Gordon's house. This was no small trauma in itself. I was filled with guilt at having left my father and brothers, but intensely saddened by having to leave my mother. I felt like a Ping-Pong ball rocketing back and forth in the game my parents seemed to be playing with one another. So it was, at the age of twelve, I was whisked back to New York to live with my father and brothers. And it was then that I first developed the feeling that everything that happened to me would always be out of my control.

I did not see my mother again for seven years. During that time, I had several asthma attacks necessitating Adrenalin shots. There is no question in my mind that the emotional climate I was forced to endure in those years contributed mightily to my having asthma and to the increasing severity of my allergy attacks.

At the age of nineteen I encouraged a reconciliation between my parents, and the family began to communicate again. I often wonder whether I would have developed asthma at all if they had found a way to stay together and battle out their differences in a more constructive way.

Around this time I got a job working as social director and master of ceremonies at a resort hotel in the Catskill Mountains. The pressure of holding down such a big responsibility finally got to me near the end of the summer season and my asthma reappeared with a vengeance. The spasm was so severe that I had to spend a week in bed. Another reason I had the spasm then (just before Labor Day) is that fall is a heavy allergy season for me. Obviously, it was the combination of emotional pressure and a potent allergy-producing climatic condition that brought me down.

My days in the hotel started promptly at nine A.M. and ended at two or three in the morning, six days a week. The seventh day was mercifully over at eight in the evening.

The first activity in the morning was usually Simon Says for the women. An hour or so later I would organize some other event in which everyone could participate until lunch at one o'clock. After lunch I would run a feeble imitation of water polo for the oldsters and start cha-cha lessons at poolside at three o'clock. For the younger guests there was softball or basketball until dinner. I was expected to run all these activities and make sure that everyone was having a good time throughout the day. That meant making jokes and generally being at everyone's disposal. This job is known as *tummler* in Yiddish jargon. Roughly translated, it means organizer, clown, kidder, or life of the party. Needless to say, it was a tall order for an inexperienced nineteen-year-old with a fully developed perfectionist bent.

After dinner I would open the casino, as it was called, and the evening's program would begin. On weeknights the guests would dance to the music of the hotel band (four student musicians who were working their way through college), play bingo with me as announcer, or be entertained by a ragtag show of sorts that I would improvise. These shows usually consisted of three or four songs sung by me or anyone else I could find who could carry a tune, plus skits or parodies of television commercials. Whoever I could press into service became an instant entertainer. Happily, it wasn't all grim. Among the hotel guests there occasionally was a talented person or two. I also found talent from among the neighboring Woodridge townies and service people who catered to the hotel.

One of my victims was a willing and extraordinarily talented counselor whom we called Mook. Mook and I frequently satirized the Temp-Tee Cream Cheese and Tip Top Lady Bread commercials. I guess it was pretty good training. I have since done twenty-five movies and Mook has become one of the most popular comedians in the nation, now using his other name, Robert Klein.

On Fridays and Saturdays the hotel would present two or three professional acts: a singer, a comic, and/or a dance act. This was a more formal show, but no less work for me since I was the master of ceremonies. I had to conduct rehearsals of the act's music charts and work out my introductions for the evening.

After activities in the casino died down and the last couple left the dance floor I would close the casino for the night, walk over to the hotel lobby, and talk and joke or *shmooze* with the remaining night-owl guests until two or three in the morning.

At that point, I would drag myself to my tiny room to get five hours of sleep or, if I had a date, stay up most of the night in a desperate attempt to have some life of my own. Needless to say, these are perfect conditions for the production of ill health. To this day I have never worked harder at any job I have ever had. All this, and fifty dollars a week.

My asthma remained quiet for the next six years except for several short-lived episodes for which I did not need treatment. But in 1965 asthma and I were reacquainted dramatically. Or musically, if you prefer. I was about to make my Broadway debut in a show called *Bajour*. It was a big, lavish musical starring Chita Rivera, Herschel Bernardi, Nancy Dussault, Robert Burr, and Herb Edelman. When I joined the cast I could hardly have imagined the powerful effect Burr and Edelman would have on the rest of my life.

It was a wonderful beginning. I had auditioned only at the finals due to my acquaintanceship with Lehman Engel, the musical director of the show and my former teacher. I was accepted and eventually, during rehearsals, was made understudy to Burr, the romantic lead. Everything was rosy. I envisioned this as the beginning of a long and illustrious musical career.

But as rehearsals progressed, I began to experience again my old breathing difficulties. Since this was an important first step in my career, I became anxious about being fired for not being able to sing the high notes required by my chorus and understudy roles. As I am sure you know, bronchitis and asthma have a marked effect on the sound of one's voice. In the case of a singer, it can end a career by shortening his or her range and phrasing capabilities. This anxiety increased as the out-of-town opening night drew near. I started taking Tedral four times daily with some relief, but my singing and the small amount of dancing required of me were seriously affected. My natural voice is high pitched (tenor), but over the period of six weeks, my upper register disappeared almost entirely. The tenor must have a B flat; I could hardly croak out a G (one and one half notes lower).

While in Boston I saw a doctor who recognized the severity of my condition and prescribed cortisone in addition to the Tedral I was already taking. The spasm was partially relieved, but the attendant bronchitis remained.

I didn't know what cortisone was. The doctor prescribed; I obeyed. But shortly thereafter I began to experience emotional symptoms that were completely new to me. For the first time in my life I became moody and suspicious. I began to have paranoid thoughts about the other members of the cast and felt as if I were ringed with enemies.

In retrospect it's clear to me that my personality, which had been gregarious and trusting, underwent a significant and detrimental change. I thought constantly of quitting the show. Bitterness and powerful negative impulses became a regular part of my emotional vocabulary. On the physical side, I was still unable to engage in rigorous exercise without getting into serious breathing difficulty.

One afternoon during the Boston tryout, while the rest of the company was rehearsing onstage, I found myself in conversation with Burr and Edelman in the lobby. I casually remarked that I had a problem with asthma. Herb said just as casually, "Oh, that can be cured." Burr said, "Oh, sure. Absolutely." You can well imagine my reaction. I must have said something like "C'mon. I've had it all my life. What are you guys talking about?"

They showed me. In less than an hour they taught me

the breathing exercises that would cure me and change the rest of my life. After explaining that these were yoga exercises specifically created for the alleviation of asthma, they took me through the exercises one by one. In the space of an hour they worked at removing my inefficient methods of respiration and replaced them with the exercises which form the bulk of the attack on asthma described in the first part of this book.

I felt better almost immediately. I thanked them both and was so exhilarated that I repeated the exercises that night for a period of forty-five minutes. I must note here that even though I was an asthmatic, I had been in the habit of vigorous physical workouts on a daily basis (I still am, but I substitute tennis now), so I was capable of doing much more than the average sedentary person. As strenuous as the exercises were, I felt stronger the longer I did them. Even more significant was that I only felt the need for two Tedral pills that day. Filled with optimism, I abandoned the cortisone immediately (if you are on cortisone presently, don't follow my example—it could be dangerous without the advice of your doctor) and spent a very restful night.

When I awoke the next morning I was astonished to find that I had no spasm whatsoever. Apart from the bronchitis, which felt like a slight chest cold, my breathing was completely free. For the first time in months I breathed like a normal person. I immediately did my exercises again for about an hour, had breakfast, and went to rehearsal in a wonderful frame of mind. Once more, Herb and Bob assured me that I would never have asthma again if I kept up the regimen. I kept it up faithfully for the next three months and by then the bronchitis had completely disappeared. I was so enthused about the system that I would practice breathing in my new way while walking on the street, driving a car, anywhere and everywhere.

My voice returned with its upper register intact, but still bearing insidious effects of my long affliction. For even though my symptoms were cured, it was to take another sixteen years before the fear of asthma would release its grip on my vocal and respiratory apparatus. From a lifetime of breathing difficulty I was in the habit of tightening my larynx while singing, due to a fear of running out of air. I was so much in the habit of gasping that even when singing something easy my voice would become pushed and tense. A voice teacher remarked once that when I sang he could see real terror in my eyes. I was only saved from this nervous breathing when a dear friend (Leonard D'John—a distance swimming champion) was trying to improve my swimming technique. He had noticed that I was not loose in the water and was at a loss to understand why I could not breathe in rhythm. With each stroke I would try to immerse my head in the water and take the breath when I came up, but within a few seconds I became panicky and would have to stop. The only way I could swim was to take huge breaths and keep my head under for ten feet or so, or swim with my head totally out of the water.

I explained to him that I could sense a real fear of being out of breath even though my lung capacity had become very large due to my years of breathing exercises. He then taught me a technique he had learned in his own training: While I held on to the ladder at the side of the pool, he instructed me to inhale naturally, immerse my head completely, and exhale slowly while counting the seconds. At first, all I could manage was six or seven seconds. But with practice, I was able to take a large breath, submerge three or four feet, and exhale up to the count of fifty-two. It was a liberating exercise.

I tried again to swim while breathing after each stroke and found that I could swim the entire length of the pool in this manner. Within a few days I applied this new ability to my singing with dramatic results. I would like to think that I will always be open to learning new ways to do things better.

One thing I know; I have always been a diehard. Had I given up my dream of becoming an operatic tenor, I never would have made my debut at age forty-two, singing six performances of *Die Fledermaus* with the Seattle Opera Association. I would never have become a proficient tennis player or learned to write advertising copy or play the piano reasonably well.

Or defeated my own asthma so that I could write this book!

Now, whenever I feel I'm getting tight while singing, I remind myself that there will always be a residual fear, but that through knowledge, a certain amount of courage, and constant application, I will be able to control the fear.

That goes for you too (whether you sing or not). In a certain sense, you must begin to take charge. No longer be dependent on inhalers, geography, climate, or any other external. By treating the problem from within, you will be able to avoid the side effects from externally induced and potentially dangerous treatments. For your own doctor will tell you that even with the most powerful weapons in the medical armamentarium, the most one can usually hope for is a depressant effect on the *symptoms* of asthma.

This is not to the discredit of the medical profession. Doctors save a great many asthmatics' lives. And thousands of dedicated physicians are treating asthma, hoping through research to find a cure for it. At this point, let me, as a notorious ex-president used to say, make this perfectly clear: I have nothing against doctors! My oldest brother is a psychiatrist, my cousin a gynecologist, my nieces and nephews all seem to be becoming doctors, and I number several doctors among my dearest friends. It is my hope that the regimen I am sharing with you, you will someday share with your doctor.

CHAPTER V

Michael's Asthma

As every father knows, there is nothing more wounding than the illness of his children. But if one feels helplessness and pain while rushing them to emergency rooms for stitches or a fever, watching your child nearly choke to death from a severe asthma attack is nothing short of a waking nightmare.

My son's first asthma attack was three years ago. I'd like to share the experience with you.

Michael was three years old then and the very picture of health. A charming, bright little boy, his energy was boundless, his spirit indomitable. He had never had allergies; even his colds were of short duration.

I was studying an opera score in my New York studio one Saturday afternoon when I got a call from my wife, Lorraine. She was worried because Michael was acting strangely and had vomited. His face was puffy and he complained that he couldn't breathe. Lorraine thought it was asthma. I knew that he had had some slight sneezing and congestion in the nose for a few days, but I thought it was nothing serious. Still, I made the half-hour trip to our house in New Jersey in twenty minutes.

He was sitting in the backyard, sort of slumped over, and looking very weak. For some reason, I couldn't accept the possibility that he might be having an asthma attack. Perhaps my guilt that I had passed this awful thing on to him made me reject the idea. I said, "No, he's sick but it's not asthma."

But it wasn't long before we both knew that a serious crisis was at hand. We called his doctor, who was out but whose service gave us the number of his cover. We called him and described Michael's condition. He told us to rush him right over. We bundled him into the car, Lorraine at the wheel and Mike in my lap as we almost flew the several miles to the doctor's office. In this time I saw Mike's eyes roll back into his head and I became terrified that we would lose him before reaching the doctor.

After what seemed an eternity, we arrived at the office. The doctor took him right into the examining room and listened to his chest. At this point Mike seemed ready to pass out. Truly alarmed, the doctor told us that he could hear nothing in Mike's right lung and thought it might be collapsed. "If he aspirates his vomit this could be very bad," he said.

He gave Mike a shot of Adrenalin and told us to watch him very carefully. He left the room to attend his other patients. We waited, terrified that Mike would vomit. In the next twenty minutes I experienced emotions I could never record. We fought to hide our tears so as not to frighten our son, and we prayed to God to save him. But Mike did not improve, and our terror mounted.

The doctor came in, listened again, and said, "The lung

is still blocked. But before we take him to the hospital, let's try another shot of Adrenalin." He did. Lorraine, the doctor, and I watched and waited five more minutes. He listened again and said he could hear air in the lung again. The lung was not collapsed, as he had feared. Michael perked up a bit. The doctor gave us prescriptions to fill. We thanked him (we'll thank him forever) and left for home.

After taking the medicines Mike seemed a good deal better, but still somewhat labored in his breathing. It was then that I began to teach him the breathing exercises that had cured me. It was a difficult task. A three-year-old boy obviously can't have the same grasp of his condition or the learning capacity that an adult has. But I knew I had to do something very soon and very definitely.

It was decided that I should sleep next to him that night in case another emergency should arise. After his bedtime story, I made it clear that he was to wake me if he had difficulty of any kind. He seemed comforted and we both drifted off.

He woke me at two in the morning, breathing spasmodically.

Games with Mike

Again I tried to teach him the exercises, but to no avail. I don't know how at that moment I came up with the idea of putting the exercises into the framework of play. I'm not good at manipulating people's behavior because when I want someone to do something I'm usually too direct. But my fear for Mike prompted some hidden resourcefulness. Out of nowhere, I pretended that my five fingers were birthday candles and said, "Wouldn't it be nice if you could blow them out, one by one?" I was of course aware that he loved to blow out the matches I used to light my pipe or cigars. And so we began to play Birthday Party. I would sing the song and he would blow out the candles. We did this for about ten minutes and he never tired of the game. It put him in a good mood even though his breathing remained labored for another hour or so. He was very talkative and not the least bit sleepy. As long as he was feeling reasonably cheerful, I assumed his condition would probably not worsen.

There followed every other kind of game that I could come up with that night. I made my hands into the shape of a bird, interlocking the thumbs, and talking in the voice of a little bird that was too weak to fly. I pleaded with my favorite little friend Michael to help me become airborne again by blowing air under my "wings." This also worked well. His nurturant instincts came into the game and it gave him a feeling of accomplishment to be able to help the little bird fly again. Each time Mike would get the bird into the air, the bird would give thanks as it flew away into the imaginary horizon.

When this game lost its freshness, I remembered that Mike was fascinated with the fires we had made together the winter before. He would gather the kindling from the backyard to help me get it going and would sit in front of the fireplace for hours, just watching it blaze. With this in mind, I put my hands together, interlocked the fingers, and pretended they were the dying embers of a once raging fire. Using the deepest, tiredest voice I could produce,

I asked my friend Mike to help me become a blaze again. He picked up the idea and blew on the "embers" time and time again. When I figured he had enlivened just enough embers not to get bored, I turned to something else.

One of Mike's favorite stories is something called "The Little Red Caboose." It saves a train from sliding down a hill. I amplified the story to encourage him to blow on the back of my hand as if it were the caboose.

By this time the successful pattern was clear and I created a number of other games using any fanciful circumstance I could think up to make him use his lung power.

It was gratifying to watch Mike that night. It gave me a lasting respect for his indomitable spirit and tender humanitarian instincts. Recognizing his need to help the little bird, the fading embers, and the little red caboose brought something into focus for me about the true nature of heroism. It was natural for him to rescue creatures and objects with which he could identify. It is probably natural and necessary for all of us.

Mike had a lot to talk about that night, and though my patience usually thins after a few minutes, I would have been glad to listen for days on end knowing how helpful it was for him. Finally, around five-thirty he became sleepy and drifted off. I said a silent prayer of thanks and slept immediately.

The next night was a carbon copy of the first. He woke again at two A.M. and we talked and played our way through the small hours.

That brought us to Monday. We took him to his regular doctor. He recommended an allergist who promptly put Mike on Slo-phyllin, Metaprel, penicillin, and a cortisone derivative. That afternoon we became aware of the devastating side effects of the cortisone.

Mike's eyes became sunken, with dilated pupils. He became frenetic, emotionally volatile. For a while we were afraid he would hurt himself with the sheer wildness of his behavior.

Within a day or two the spasm was gone. I had to leave on a business trip for a week, but Lorraine moved Mike into our bedroom and kept up the regimen day and night while I was gone. In that time she developed a number of new exercises with Mike. For instance, she would light a real candle and have him blow it out at varying distances. She would dampen a cloth and ask him to pressure it enough with his breath to lift it horizontally. I stayed in close touch several times a day by phone. When I returned he was well enough to be able to sleep alone again, though his emotional state was still upsetting to us.

After two weeks we took him back to the allergist, who seemed surprised to see him doing so well. He took him off all medication. Even though the crisis was over, we continued the exercise/play for six or seven weeks.

Five months later, after spending an asthma-free summer, he began to show again the telltale symptoms that had signaled his first attack. His eyelids began to swell, his face was puffy and covered with tiny bumps, and he developed a bronchitic cough. But this time we were ready.

We brought him to the allergist again. He told us that because we had caught it early, there would be no need for cortisone. We took him home, gave him the prescribed Tedral elixir, and moved him into our bedroom for a few days.

For the next several weeks, we devoted ourselves to the

alleviation of this second near-asthmatic attack. Within days the bronchitis began to ease. We took him off the Tedral and maintained only a minimal dose of antihistamine. His allergic symptoms remained for a few more weeks, but he had no trouble breathing and the bronchitis disappeared shortly thereafter.

For me, this was proof positive that Michael had conquered his asthma. He has since been free of any asthma symptoms for two and a half years, though in that time he has had chest colds and allergy problems (sniffling and sneezing). This is remarkable since, as every asthmatic knows, a chest cold or allergic reaction is frequently the beginning of another asthmatic episode.

With this in mind we take nothing for granted. As soon as he shows the slightest sign of a stuffy nose, we begin a strong program of the exercise/play. Lorraine drops other activities and devotes her time and attention to Mike. We suspect he likes that part of the treatment best, but it has not, at least so far, encouraged him to become sick again. Even when he is well, I try not to let more than a few days go by without doing at least a few exercises with him.

During these sessions I always check to see if he is taking a breath deep in the lungs and using the diaphragm correctly. If not, I put my hands under his ribs and practice with him. I also take care to do all this with a spirit of fun and adventure. A child will take his behavioral cues from Mommy and Daddy. If you are grim and desperate, the game is over before it begins. But if you decide that asthma is absolutely defeatable, that together you can, and must, come up with the solution, your child will go along. There are also times when you have to insist, even if it means no dessert or, heaven help us, no cartoons on Saturday morning.

In other words, it must become important enough to you to make sacrifices, strain your creativity and patience to the breaking point, and exercise parental prerogatives strongly, even if you have raised your child in a liberal way. I disdain spanking my children except in extreme cases, am lenient (overly so, sometimes), but I let nothing stand in my way when it comes to making sure he doesn't get asthma again.

CHAPTER VI

More Games

The Cambini Special

There is a bedtime story Lorraine created called the "Cambini Special." It was always one of Mike's favorites so I decided to use it. In the voice of a train track announcer I act out the story of a train that leaves Grand Central Station, complete with names of all the intended cities. By the time I say, "All aboard," Mike begins to huff and puff as if he were the engine. As the train progresses, it picks up speed, as does the rhythm of his breathing. I say things like "We are now passing over the great plains of Nebraska. To your right you will see the Grand Canyon. Now passing through Denver, Phoenix, Philadelphia." (My geographical accuracy isn't too dependable.) "The last hurdle is the Rocky Mountains." I make the sound of the train whistle and exhort Mike to blow as hard as he can to pull that train, that big, black engine, over the mountains. When he has done enough, the game is over and I say, "We have now arrived at Los Angeles Station. Thank you for traveling on the Cambini Special."

He enjoys this game so much, he often asks to do it, sometimes doing part of the narration himself.

Power Boy and Asthma Man

This game is more physical and involves what most boys like to do: act out the roles of superheroes and supervillains. It came about in an interesting manner.

Much of Mike's free time is spent as a knight in his toy plastic armor, jousting with other imaginary knights. He also went through an intense Spiderman phase, shooting out webs to ensnare bad guys.

Wrestling is fun for him too (bad guys or good guys will do). When I'm not home he often pins his mother and sisters to the mat to establish his male "superiority" (they have to cooperate, of course).

One day after we had done some breathing exercises together, we began to wrestle and Mike became Spiderman. As we tussled on the rug, I began to improvise the role of a supervillain. I broke loose and took an awesome pose. Kneeling down with arms outstretched, fingers pointed downward, I grandly announced that I was Asthma Man. Mike took the hint right away and literally began to blow me down. I cried out in mock horror that I didn't mean it and he shouldn't hurt me or I wouldn't be able to make all the other little children sick anymore. He pounced on me, huffing and puffing with all his strength. But as soon as I was defeated, I metamorphosed into

Bronchitis Man and suggested that Mike should become Power Boy. In my new character, I told Mike that I "could help him with his breathing, that he should breathe high in the chest." He shouted back that his daddy had taught him "the right way, down here" (indicating his diaphragm and breathing forcefully in and out). I snarled back that his daddy was a no-good liar. That really got him going. He jumped all over me and "defeated" me again.

At this point I became my final villain by proclaiming myself Sick Lungs Man. I boasted that only one thing could defeat me: the Bellows (I had taught this exercise to Mike sometime before, and though he didn't grasp the entire concept, he was able to execute a reasonable version of it). In response, Mike announced proudly that he knew the Bellows and that he was now . . . Superman. As he did his version of the Bellows, I gasped and dropped to the rug, finished off for good.

We must have done this one at least a hundred times at bedtimes. I never cease to be amazed at how well he understands the nature of the game and how imaginative a person he really is. But this is true of most children. Their most valuable asset is their imagination and their faith in imaginary circumstances. The trick for the parents of an asthmatic is to help put the child's potent fantasy life to work for the child.

This approach has been marvelously effective for us because the breathing exercises are hard work and most people, young or old, would rather play than work. In my experience with Mike and other children, without the play aspect, the exercises would be intolerable.

* * *

Some might say that this game, combative in nature as it is, might tend to encourage aggressive tendencies in a child. I would agree completely. But we must remember that an asthmatic child is often passive in temperament. A strong dose of assertiveness training is all to the good, perhaps indispensable, if we are to help rid the child of asthma.

There is no advantage for it to be said about a child that he or she "wouldn't hurt a fly." There are times when all of us must do battle of some kind, whether it be actual or psychological. When this battle is waged in the defense of others, it isolates and develops the very essence of heroism, which, when you think about it, is not a bad thing.

Remember while doing this exercise with your child that it is also an opportunity for both of you to share a healthy form of affection. When wrestling with him, I take care to give Mike a good scrap but never to hurt him and, by the end of the game, I see to it that he always defeats my supervillain.

PART III

Sharing the Exercises

CHAPTER VII

Case Histories

In the last twenty years I have been able to share what I have learned with several hundred others. Seeing people released from the tyranny of asthma has been one of the most gratifying experiences of my life.

Chris

Chris is a sixteen-year-old boy who had required several trips to the hospital for acute asthma attacks. His father, Charles Garbaccio, and mother, Heather, are friends of our family and, ironically, Charles is a prominent physician, specializing in plastic surgery. The boy's situation came to my attention when, at a party, someone mentioned that I was writing a book about asthma. Charles and Heather were very interested, so I invited the family over in order to teach Chris the exercises. I learned that the asthma had interfered seriously with his high school soccer career. He often had to be benched several times during a game.

I started as I always do by asking him to take a deep breath. Predictably, he heaved his chest up high while taking a shallow breath. I noticed that his voice was hollow (most asthmatics sound that way). He had a stuffy nose and I could hear the congestion in his chest when he coughed; the dry unproductive cough of the asthmatic.

I put him through the exercises, taking great care that he understood everything every step of the way. He grasped the concept quickly, but found the coordination difficult at first. But he was so determined that he pushed abnormally hard in a muscular way. I began to worry that he might go into spasm right there; but after all, there was a doctor in the house. After about twenty minutes he coughed a few more times, but this time with a difference. We could all hear him loosening up in the chest. I asked him if he felt any better. He smiled for the first time since he had come into the room and said, "Yeah. It feels good."

By now, partly because of his physical exertion and partly because his body was beginning to get some badly needed oxygen, his facial color had noticeably begun to change. Charles agreed that the coloring was in part due to the sudden oxygenation of Chris's body. So far, so good. Medical affirmation.

It got better. So encouraged was Charles that he suggested, insisted might be the better word, that we go through the exercises again. Chris agreed and we did just that. Fifteen minutes later we were all convinced that Chris, though totally exhausted, had successfully learned them.

A few days later, Heather called to say that Chris had

scored three goals in his last game and was doing the exercises twice daily.

It's been a year since he started and there has been no asthma.

The Sound Man's Son

Two years ago, while doing a movie in Los Angeles called *Off the Wall,* I learned that the sound engineer's son had asthma. I invited them over. The boy was thirteen, breathing with considerable difficulty, and had been restricted athletically. He too had been a good athlete before the asthma forced him off the baseball field.

I also recognized that his father was an asthmatic type. When I asked him, he confirmed that he occasionally got attacks as well. Within a half hour, father and son left, but not until they both had learned the exercises. Three hours later they called to say that the boy was breathing freely for the first time in six months.

Elaine

I first heard about Elaine when I ran into an internist friend at a barbershop in Manhattan. We hadn't seen one another in about ten years, and after both of us remarked how well the other looked, Jack mentioned that his son had read about my involvement with a treatment for asthma. He then told me about his wife, Elaine, who was on high doses of Prednisone and that he was deeply concerned about the growing side effects.

She had been getting worse and worse over the past four years. The best doctors available had treated her, but her condition would improve slightly and only for short intervals. I told Jack that although I couldn't guarantee she would be cured, I was sure that I could help her to some degree and would call her soon.

Several days later, when my wife and I were at a party at the home of Dr. Charles Garbaccio (the plastic surgeon), I became involved in a discussion about asthma. It began by my remarking how well his son Chris looked. Now I must tell you that after two drinks, I am willing to discuss anything with anyone. On this particular night, I had chosen to lecture at length on the subject of asthma with Mac Borg, the owner of *The Bergen Record,* a large newspaper in our county. I said, with all the authority of a visiting bishop, something like "Doctors haven't found the cure to this disease because it isn't a disease at all." It turned out to be an especially ill-advised pronunciamento since, as I later learned, the place was wall-to-wall with doctors.

Nor was my punishment long delayed. Mac, the publisher, leaned over to a fellow standing nearby and, in a voice more suited to an auctioneer imploring a final bid, said, "This guy says you guys don't know much about asthma!" Back shot the reply, "Nothing at all!" Something told me that I had cast a fateful die and I rushed to recover the situation by introducing myself and trying to backtrack. Turns out the fellow was Jim Smith, one of the most prominent lung specialists in the world and the president of the New York chapter of the Lung Association of America.

His attitude was ironic but tolerant and instead of a war, we began to engage in a fruitful talk about the subject. While explaining my theories and sharing some of my experiences, he informed me that he knew very well that inhaling through the nose was of critical importance to asthmatics since mouth breathing closes the throat.

I was grateful that this eminent physician was genuinely interested in what I had to say. He suggested that we test out my program with some of his more seriously afflicted patients and started to tell me about the wife of a colleague who had been on megadoses of Prednisone. Small world, eh?

We both felt that it was almost too stunning a coincidence. He suggested we should not tell Elaine that we had talked but that I should call her and proceed to teach her the exercises.

A few days later I met with Elaine at Jack's office. One could see at a glance that this attractive woman was suffering greatly from cortisone side effects.

I went through the program with her for about forty-five minutes. It seemed to have an immediate effect. She coughed productively at least eight times and I left the office in the highest of spirits.

The following week, when I called to set up another appointment with Elaine, Jack told me that she had had a very bad weekend. I was chagrined, to say the least, but we scheduled the time anyway.

At this session she told me that after two days of doing the exercises faithfully, she had so improved that she lowered her dose of Prednisone by 25 percent. The following day the breathing difficulty returned in force.

I asked her to show me how she had been doing the exercises. She sat on a chair and performed the seated portion flawlessly. I became more disheartened but asked her to go on and show me the Bellows. She did so, and I saw at once that her approach to the exercise was incomplete. As she leaned forward to begin, she expressed almost no air at all. As she straightened up, I could see very little air coming in; and as she pushed forward, there was, of course, only that small amount of air to be forced out.

I showed her what she had to do and had her repeat it two more times. She coughed productively again. I told her that despite her comprehension and enthusiasm, her body was not yet in condition to reduce any medication.

Three weeks later, with her doctor's approval, she lowered her dosage by one third and was feeling much improved.

Harriet

Several months ago, my wife, Lorraine, mentioned that a lovely woman with whom she did volunteer work at church had severe asthma. It was a familiar story. Numerous crises, hospital visits, heavy doses of cortisone with its frightening side effects (in her case, bone fractures and muscle deterioration in her back), further complicated by the fact that she is seventy-four years old and has suffered with asthma all her life.

At first sight I was charmed by Harriet. She was bright,

looked young for her years, and was obviously a person who cared about herself. Even though I knew her age would be a negative factor, I could tell she had spirit and I was anxious to begin working with her.

Because of her age, I proceeded cautiously. She was quick to understand the principles involved, but had trouble maintaining a strong lip pressure. Also, from years of high "chest" breathing, her clavicles and pectoral structure were so pushed out, it was difficult for her to take a deep breath using the diaphragm muscle fully stretched. Needless to say, after all those years of disuse, her diaphragm was very weak.

Though I didn't show it, I was disappointed, for even after a half hour of working together, there was no productive cough. She told me she felt a little better, but I was not encouraged. I suggested she do her exercises faithfully, gave her my usual pep talk, and asked her to return the following week.

Frankly, at that point, I didn't think the program would be a success with her because of her long asthmatic history and advanced age. I felt that she would never be able to develop the necessary strength to reverse the damage a lifetime of labored breathing had produced.

She came to the house the following Friday. As I had expected, there hadn't been much progress, if any at all. I went through the complete program again. She did seem to grasp more of it this time and even managed a couple of slightly productive coughs before we were finished. But inwardly, I felt it was too little, too late. I wished her luck and asked her to call me in a month. After she left I told Lorraine that it was hopeless. This poor lady had been sick too many years for me or anyone else to turn the tide.

Three weeks later, I found out how wrong I had been. Turns out she got so much better that a few days after our second session she lowered her cortisone dose by one third (her doctor allowed it), and at the time of this writing (four weeks later), she is doing her exercises sedulously and feeling much better while still on that lowered dose.

To me, this woman is nothing less than a heroine. At a time in life when most people are ready to abandon everything for the rocking chair, Harriet is in there pitching, fighting her asthma, doing good works for her church and community, and being an example of courage that people half her age would do well to emulate.

John's Son

During the making of the movie *That Championship Season,* Martin Sheen and I became good friends. As is customary on the set of a movie, there are often long stretches of waiting before the actors are required in front of the camera to film the next take. For me, these times were filled with chess, tennis, or just talk. Since asthma is never far from my thoughts and Martin is a yoga practitioner, we talked often about the healthful aspects of yoga breathing techniques.

One day, several months after the filming was completed, I got a call from Martin in California. He told me that a friend of his, John, was distressed by the fact that his son was suffering a severe asthma attack for the second time. The boy was not yet three and had already undergone heavy medical treatment, including cortisone therapy. Martin asked if I would call his friend and see if I could help in any way.

At the sound of John's voice on the telephone, I could tell that his son was in a crisis. It recalled to me the desperation I had felt when Michael had been so ill.

I explained that it would be difficult to help since we lived at opposite ends of the country but that I would try to share the information as best I could over the phone. I recounted my experiences with Michael in great detail and stressed the importance of the game factor. It was frustrating to me since I knew there was no substitute for seeing the child and working with him to ensure that he learn and accept the exercise/games in toto. We exchanged goodbyes and vowed to keep in touch.

A year passed and, though from time to time I wondered how the boy was doing, I never seemed to have the time to call and follow up.

Three days ago, under pressure of meeting the deadline for this book, I called to find out the result of my telephone "treatment."

Nothing could have been more gratifying. John told me that his son had quickly recovered from the terrible attack he had sustained back at the time of our phone call. He had had one more very slight episode a few months later where the doctor needed only to prescribe an antibiotic to clear it up, and there had been no asthma at all since that time.

He told me how he created the character of Captain Asthma for his son to blow across the room. How he imitated Marcel Marceau in a windstorm to his son's total delight. He observed that the wonderful mood the game engendered in him also seemed to have a healing effect. And he told me how grateful he was for what I had shared with him on the phone a year ago.

I asked him if he would mind my including this story in the book. He said he would be honored and happy to if I thought it would help.

I literally shouted to everyone in the house after hanging up the phone. "Thank God! John's son is healthy again."

John Ritter, the great television star, is also a great father.

Ron, the Cigar Store Man

One of the vices I enjoy with impunity since I banished my asthma is occasionally to smoke a good cigar. I have them aged and keep them at a tobacconist's shop in midtown Manhattan. On one of my visits there about six months ago, I noticed that Ron, the man in charge of the humidifier, sounded congested and hollow-voiced. As you might imagine, I have become very sensitive to the sound of the asthmatic voice.

I asked him if he had asthma. He said he did from time to time. I asked him to take a large breath. As I expected, the chest went up, the wheeze became audible, and the hopeless look on his face became more marked.

I asked him if he knew where his lungs were. He told me he did and pointed directly to the middle of his chest. Trying not to be too obnoxious, I proceeded to correct his misapprehension. Then I showed him the exercises. He seemed a little better, but I could tell he had reservations.

It was his opinion, and this is a common one, that his affliction was purely psychological. I suggested that he was partly right, that the asthma was his body's method of dealing with allergies and stress. He lit my cigar, I wished him luck and went on my way.

Just today, I went back to the shop to pick up a box of my cigars and found him breathing perfectly, without the slightest trace of asthma or bronchitis. I asked him if he had been doing the exercises. By the look on his face I could tell they had not become a major part of his life. He replied, guiltily, that he had only done them for a week. I offered that that had obviously been enough. But, stubborn to the end, he insisted that his cure was "psychological" because once he recognized that he had created the condition, *he* was the one who could remove it. I had to agree with that too.

But as I was leaving, he shot out, "Besides, once I realized where my lungs were, that made a difference."

The Meeting

Some time ago, an item appeared in Earl Wilson's newspaper column that I was writing a book on defeating asthma. More than five hundred letters poured in to the William Morrow offices from all over the country asking for information about my "method."

I was nonplussed. As I read them I was almost overcome by the heartbreaking stories in those letters. The children who didn't grow, the repeated hospital crises, the otherwise normal people who had become near invalids from their tragic asthmatic afflictions.

I decided that something had to be done, so I sent out a form letter inviting all who could come to a meeting that I would hold in New York City. I got hundreds of responses saying that they would attend. I hired a hall and within a few weeks the meeting came about.

It turned out to be an incredible experience. People of every description showed up. The age range was from three to over eighty. The hall was so filled that there weren't enough chairs for everybody, so most of the younger ones had to sit on the floor.

I began by telling of my experiences and my approach to the problem. Then, one by one, I began to work individually, taking each person through the floor and chair portions of the exercises. The experience began to take on the character of a revival meeting as, one by one, each person in the room contributed energy and enthusiasm.

After I had worked with more than a hundred people, one woman raised her hand and asked to speak. She told us all, with tears in her eyes, that she had left the meeting to go a block away to the drugstore just a few minutes before and had realized that for the first time in years she had walked that distance without getting out of breath. Another woman, one of the first with whom I had worked, held up her inhaler, which she said she had used at least twenty times during that day, and said that she had not had to use it that evening.

The meeting lasted more than three hours. There were

lots of hugs and handshakes. At the end I was so exhausted I could hardly walk. But it was an evening I will never forget and for which I will always be grateful, for I believe that almost everyone there was helped to some degree.

CHAPTER VIII

You and Your Doctor

I am obviously not a graduate of Harvard Medical School. You know me as an actor and singer if you know me at all. Why then follow my advice on an issue that involves your most precious possession, your health?

Perhaps the most compelling reason is that with none of my suggestions will you have anything to lose except your asthma.

But it isn't my intention to replace your doctor's care. My personal experience and research are what I'm sharing with you, plus a good deal of information from some marvelous doctors who have treated me and advised me over the years. The fact is, I'm going to ask you to talk this program over with your own doctor very carefully. Assuming that you are in otherwise good health, he will most likely advise you to try the exercises. In the event that he does not, the decision will be yours. But bear in mind that he may feel you have other health problems that may be worsened by taking up this program.

I think it wise to adopt the attitude that your doctor

wants the best for you and it is in your own interest to work the problem through with his help, inspiration, and guidance. If you are on anti-asthma medication, you must continue taking it until your doctor says it is no longer necessary, that is, until you are symptom-free.

Diet

I believe proper diet can be very important in the campaign to defeat asthma even when the asthma is not associated with an identifiable allergy. You would have to search long and hard to find a professional opera singer who would even dream of drinking milk or eating chocolate on the day of a performance. This is because singers are convinced these foods cause a buildup of mucus in the body.

The eminent throat specialist Eugen Grabscheid, also known as the "singer's doctor," has been treating vocal problems for over fifty years. It is his opinion, based on the treatment of thousands of singers, that to avoid a buildup of mucus in the body one must avoid whole milk and whole milk products, red wine, chocolate, and all foods containing monosodium glutamate.

Obviously, denying yourself or your children such foods can create a major management problem. But, with a little imagination, alternatives can be found. For example, during a severe allergy season or at the onset of an asthmatic episode, use apple juice on cereal instead of milk. If you are concerned about calcium deficiency, ask your doctor about taking calcium supplements. Later, when the crisis has passed, switch to skim milk. Believe it or not, after drinking skim milk for a time, whole milk will seem too rich to you.

There are commercially available frozen desserts made with skim milk that can be served instead of ice cream and actually taste very good. Another alternative is To-futti, a product similar in texture and taste to ice cream, yet containing no dairy product whatsoever. Meringues, ices (not sherbet, which is made with milk), and gelatin with fruit are also good possibilities.

Please don't get the idea that I'm encouraging sugar intake. Far from it. My personal opinion is that by revving up the body with too much sugar, allergies may actually be worsened. It's just that it is unwise to fight all your enemies at the same time. For your children, it's next to impossible.

If you're concerned about sugar, use a substitute. Short-term use is probably not harmful and, in this case, the benefit would seem to outweigh the risk.

The culprit in red wine is a substance called tannin. I love good red wine, but in the fall I drink only white. As far as chocolate is concerned, the closest substitute is something called carob. Health-food stores stock it in nearly limitless varieties.

Specific Allergies

There are a number of people who are allergic to specific foods such as wheat or shellfish. The best way to find out if you have a specific food or environmental allergy, such as to dust, pollen, or animal dander, is to be tested either by blood analysis or the traditional scratch test. Once your doctor has pinpointed your potentially harmful allergens, you can try to take the necessary steps to avoid them.

In the case of wheat allergy, rice cakes, corn and protein breads, and corn and oat-based cereals are helpful substitutes. If you are allergic to pasta, there is a macaroni-type product made from artichoke flour that is very tasty. Of course you will defeat your own purpose if you prepare it with cheese or butter or use grated cheese on it. Instead, you can use any number of vegetables, such as broccoli or peas, with a little garlic and onion, sautéed in olive oil or margarine.

Vitamins

Take them. Don't make a religion out of them. So far, there is no evidence that vitamin therapy has a noticeable effect on asthma. I take them in moderation and we give them to Michael, but in my experience their value is primarily in promoting good overall health.

Other Allergens

Feather-filled comforters, pillows, and cushions can be dangerous to asthmatics. Give them away and replace them with nonallergenic types. The same goes for stuffed animals. Try to get your children used to rubber toys instead.

Some asthmatics are allergic to wool. Use cotton or synthetic fabrics in their place. This goes for the carpets as well.

Dust is a potent allergen and bothers a great many asthmatics. Dust everything frequently with a slightly dampened cloth and make sure to vacuum curtains and draperies on a regular schedule. It is also a good idea to invest in a good room air purifier, or attach one to your home heating or cooling system.

If you live in a cold climate, use a humidifier in the winter. Inside, heated air is too dry and can create breathing problems. If your climate is overly humid, such as it is in the southern states, mold spores can be a problem. A good way to counter this is to use a dehumidifier or air conditioner to cut down on mold spore growth.

Dogs, cats, hamsters, birds, etc., are all better suited to life on a farm than in the home of an asthmatic. We had an interesting problem with this one because our daughter Amanda had a dozen pet mice. I knew that I had to clear them out for Michael's sake, but Amanda was brokenhearted at the thought. The solution was reached when I spent several hours building an intricate mouse house out of plywood, complete with little windows and a door. I then persuaded Amanda that her brother's health was at risk and that the mice would be much happier out of our basement and in their new little house. As far as she and I know, they are still romping merrily in the woods.

By the way, if your doctor recommends them, don't be afraid to take antihistamines in allergy seasons such as spring and fall.

The Future

It is likely that asthma afflicts over one hundred million people worldwide. Its tragic effects range from slight breathing difficulty to near invalidism and premature death. Yet, there is still only scant attention paid to it by the general public.

There are fund campaigns, powerful national organizations, and telethons for such serious diseases as muscular dystrophy, multiple sclerosis, cerebral palsy, and a host of others. There has even been a traffic safety telethon. This is all to the good. Those who involve themselves in these campaigns are on the side of the angels. But for the life of me, I cannot imagine why, even allowing for the unheroic reputation asthma carries, so few seem ready to come to the rescue.

While there are organizations in existence to disseminate information about asthma and allergies, they are made up largely of health professionals. It is my dream that in the near future an organization consisting only of recovered asthmatics in every country could be launched to spread these techniques—an organization of volunteers founded solely for the purpose of one human being helping another.

Think of the value it could have. If children were spared this bullying illness at an early age, imagine the suffering these children and their families would avoid.

In Fine

Please remember that the exercises are not like penicillin or cortisone, which work independently of your will. This program is in you, produced by you, and if it's going to work, must be backed to the hilt by you.

Finally, don't give up. Push against the tide. Have determination and courage. You will prevail.

Index

Adrenalin, 17, 49
Allergens, 88–89
  animal dander, 89, 90
  dust, 89, 90
  feathers, 89–90
  pollen, 89
  scratch tests for, 89
  shellfish, 88
  wheat, 88–89
  wool, 90
Analogy of the balloon, 16–17, 23
  exercises and, 23
Animal dander, 89, 90
Antibiotics, 18, 19
Antihistamines, 18
Assertiveness, 44, 69
  children's games and, 69
Asthma:
  allergens and, 88–89
  assertiveness and, 44, 69
  balloon analogy and, 16–17, 23
  breathlessness and, 20
  chest distended by, 19
  congestion, 15

contempt by others toward asth-
    matics, 20
coronary disease and, 16
cortisone and, 18, 19, 53, 63
cure for, 16
defined, 15–17
diet and, 87–88
dignity and asthmatics, 20–21
as disorder of respiratory process,
    16
doctors and, 56–57, 86–87
drugs prescribed for, 17–18
effects of, 19–20
exercises for. *See* Exercises
fear of, 55
genetic predisposition to, 15, 44
loss of work time and, 19–20
nondisease concept, 16
organizations for, 91
physical symptoms, 20–21
as "psychosomatic," 20
psychotherapy and, 44
repression of feelings and, 43
shallow breathing pattern, 15

Index

Asthma (*continued*)
    spasms, 15, 17–19
Asthma exercises. *See* Exercises
Asthma Man and Power Boy (game
    for children), 67–69

Bajour, 52
Balloon analogy, 16–17, 23
    exercises and, 23
Bellows exercise, 30–32
Bergen Record, The, 76
Bernardi, Herschel, 52
Borg, Mac, 76
Bronchitis Man (game for children),
    68
Bronchodilators, 18, 19
Burr, Robert, 52, 53–54
    teaches exercises to author, 53–54

Calcium, 87
"Cambini Special" (game for chil-
    dren), 66–67
Caruso, Enrico, 30
Case histories, 73–85
    Chris (sixteen-year-old boy), 73–75
    Elaine, 75–78
    Harriet, 78–80
    John Ritter's son, 80–82
    the meeting, 83–85
    Ron, the cigar store man, 82–83
    sound engineer's son, 75
Chair exercises, 28–32
Chest distended by asthma, 19
Child asthmatics, 18, 63
    cortisone and, 18, 63
    See also Games for children; Sor-
        vino, Michael
Chocolate, 87, 88
Congestion, 15
Coronary disease, 16, 32
    exercises and, 32

Cortisone, 18, 19, 53, 63
    author's use of, 53
    effects on children, 18, 63

Dehumidifiers, 90
Diaphragm and exercises, 24, 25
    conscious control, 25
Diet, 87–88, 89
    calcium, 87
    chocolate, 87, 88
    milk products, 87–88
    monosodium glutamate, 87
    mucus buildup and, 87
    red wine, 87, 88
    sugar, 88
    vitamins, 89
    See also Allergens
D'John, Leonard, 55
Doctors and asthma, 56–57, 86–87
Drugs, 17–18
Dussault, Nancy, 52
Dust allergy, 89, 90

Edelman, Herb, 52, 53–54
    teaches exercises to author, 53–54
Elaine (case history), 75–78
Engel, Lehman, 52
Exercises, 22–41, 42–43
    Bellows exercise, 30–32
    chair exercises, 28–32
    clothing for, 23
    coughing sensation and, 27–28
    diaphragm and, 24, 25
    diaphragmatic breathing and, 24
    equipment for, 23
    exhalation, 25–26
    floor exercises, 23–27
    heart disease and, 32
    hyperventilation during, 29
    illustrations for, 34–41
    inhalation, 23–25

learning, 22
mirror used for, 23
"muscle memory" and, 33
persistence and, 33
pharynx and, 31
positive shouting and, 29–30
punching bag, 42–43
relaxation in breathing, 25–26
taking time to learn, 22
"Train. Don't strain," 25
variation on, 27
water consumption and, 28
when to practice, 33
See also Case histories; Games for children
Exhalation exercises, 25–26

Feather allergy, 89–90
Fledermaus, Die, 56

Games for children, 60–61, 66–69
assertiveness in, 69
Asthma Man and Power Boy, 67–69
Birthday Party, 60
"Cambini Special," 66–67
Garbaccio, Christopher (case history), 73–75
Garbaccio, Dr. Charles, 73, 74, 76
Garbaccio, Heather, 73
Genetic predisposition, 15, 44
Gordon, Mrs. ("Mother"), 47–49
Grabscheid, Dr. Eugen, 87

Harriet (case history), 78–80
Heart disease, 16, 32
exercises and, 32
Humidifiers, 90
Hyperventilation and exercises, 29

Illustrations of exercises, 34–41
Inhalation exercises, 23–25

Klein, Robert, 51

"Little Red Caboose, The," 62

Meeting for asthmatics, 83–85
Metaprel, 62
Milk products, 87–88
Monosodium glutamate, 87
Mucus buildup, 15, 87
diet and, 87

Off the Wall (film), 75
Out-of-breath feeling, 20

Penicillin, 62
Pets, 89, 90
Pharynx, 31
Physical symptoms, 20–21
Physicians. See Doctors and asthma
Pollen, 89
Positive shouting, 29–30
Power Boy and Asthma Man (game for children), 67–69
assertiveness and, 69
Prednisone, 18, 76
Psychotherapy, 44
assertiveness and, 44
genetic predisposition and, 44
Punching-bag exercise, 42–43
aggressive feelings and, 43
hitting function and, 43

Red wine, 87, 88
tannin in, 88
Relaxation in breathing, 25–26
Repression of feelings, 43
Ritter, John, 80–82
Rivera, Chita, 52

Index

Ron, the cigar store man (case history), 82–83

Scratch tests, 89
Sheen, Martin, 80
Shellfish, 88
Sick Lungs Man (game for children), 68
Skim milk, 88
Slo-phyllin, 62
Smith, Dr. Jim, 76–77
Sorvino, Amanda, 90
Sorvino, Lorraine, 19, 58–60, 63, 64, 66, 78, 79
Sorvino, Michael, 18, 58–65
    early warning symptoms of second attack, 63–64
    exercise-play program for, 64
    first asthma attack, 58–60
    games created for, 60–61
Sorvino, Paul, 18, 19, 45–57
    arranges meeting for asthmatics, 83–85
    Broadway debut of, 52–54
    at children's asthmatic center, 18
    on doctors and asthma, 56–57, 86–87
    fear of asthma after initial relief, 55
    first cortisone use, 53
    first experience with asthma, 47

learns exercises from fellow actors, 53–54
Mrs. Gordon and, 47–49
opera career of, 19
resort hotel work of, 49–52
son's asthma. *See* Sorvino, Michael
swimming-pool exercise technique, 55–56
Spasm, 15, 17–19
    Adrenalin for, 17
    drugs prescribed for, 17–18
    as overreaction, 15
    predictable course of, 17
    stress and, 17
Stress, 17
Stuffed animals, 89
Sugar, 88
Symptoms of asthma, 20–21

Tannin, 88
Tedral, 18, 52, 53
That Championship Feeling (film), 80
"Train. Don't strain," 25

Vanceril, 18
Vitamins, 89

Water consumption, 28
Wheat allergy, 88–89
Wine, red, 87
Wool allergy, 90